How to Stop Insomnia

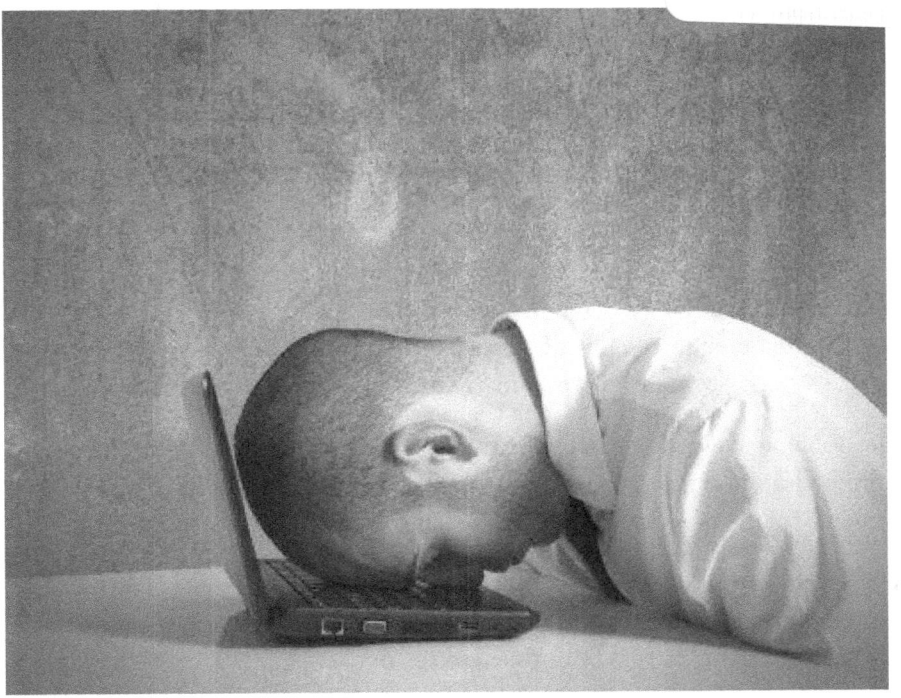

Science of Living Series

M. Usman

Mendon Cottage Books

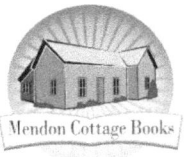

JD-Biz Publishing

Disclaimer

The information is this book is provided for informational purposes only. It is not intended to be used and medical advice or a substitute for proper medical treatment by a qualified health care provider. The information is believed to be accurate as presented based on research by the author.

The contents have not been evaluated by the U.S. Food and Drug Administration or any other Government or Health Organization and the contents in this book are not to be used to treat cure or prevent disease.

The author or publisher is not responsible for the use or safety of any diet, procedure or treatment mentioned in this book. The author or publisher is not responsible for errors or omissions that may exist.

Warning

The Book is for informational purposes only and before taking on any diet, treatment or medical procedure, it is recommended to consult with your primary health care provider.

Our books are available at

1. Amazon.com
2. Barnes and Noble
3. Itunes
4. Kobo
5. Smashwords
6. Google Play Books

Table of Contents

Introduction

Sleep habits we learn as children may play a vital role in affecting our sleep patterns as we grow. Poor sleep or lifestyle habits usually cause insomnia. Insomnia is a common sleep disorder in which you may have trouble falling asleep or staying asleep or both. According to some estimates, millions of people worldwide are living with insomnia. It not only affects your sleep but also takes away your efficacy at your day time work.

Common symptoms could be lying awake for a long time, sleeping for small periods, staying awake through the night, waking up too early or feeling as if you didn't sleep at all.

Once diagnosed with insomnia as per your medical and sleep history, your doctor may recommend a sleep study to gather the information related to your sleep and how your body responds to your sleep problems. After diagnosis, treatments related to lifestyle changes, counseling, and medicines may be recommended.

Insomnia is very well curable but it needs to be managed and kept under control by learning to take things as they are. With this stressful lifestyle, it's important to learn some of the relaxation techniques to detoxify ourselves and to keep such stress related problems at par.

Chapter #1: What is Insomnia and Types of Insomnia

Insomnia:

Insomnia is when a person faces difficulty in initiating or/and maintaining a sound sleep. It occurs due to inadequate quantity or quality of sleep. It may be natural to have a night or two of disturbed sleep due to health conditions, change of environment, change of routine, change of place, etc but if the same sleepiness nights occur for more than a week, it may require some medical attention.

Types of Insomnia:

Though there is no standard demarcation in classifying Insomnia under various types but on a general note, it is classified in three categories based on duration of the problem.

❖ **Transient Insomnia:** Symptoms lasting from a couple of days to a week.

❖ **Short Term Insomnia:** It is also known as acute Insomnia. Here the symptoms persist from a week to a month.

❖ **Chronic Insomnia:** When the symptoms persist for months, it results into chronic Insomnia. As per health experts, majority of chronic insomnia symptoms are side effects of some other problem.

Insomnia is not age dependent, it can affect anyone. Among adults, women are more affected by Insomnia than men. It is more common in people under stress, and people dealing with some medical or health problems like depression, anxiety, obesity, poor immune system, memory problems, etc.

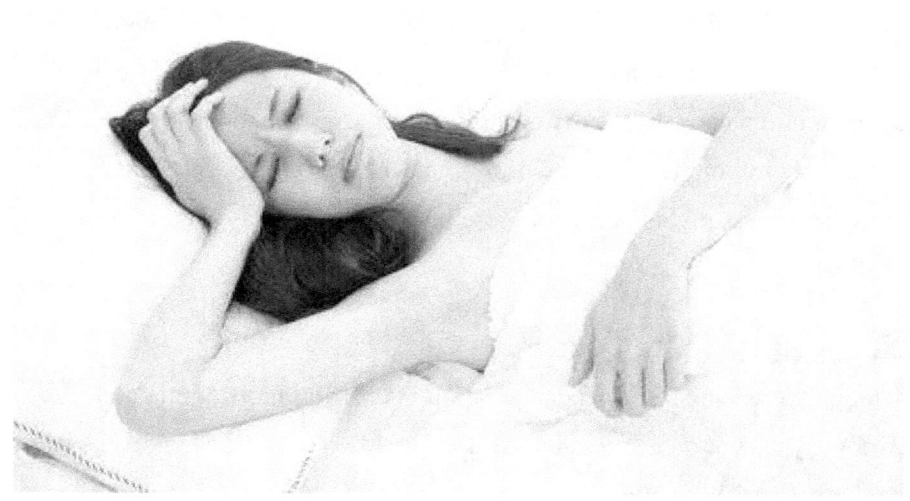

Symptoms and Causes

Chapter #2: Causes of Insomnia

Insomnia may be caused by different factors that could be physical, medical, situational, or psychological.

Causes of transient and Acute or short term Insomnia are almost similar. These may include:

- ❖ Change in working hours
- ❖ Uncomfortable bedroom temperature (too hot or too cool)
- ❖ Jet lag
- ❖ Excessive or unpleasant sounds near the bedroom
- ❖ Medical Condition like fever, cold and congestion, diarrhea, cough, breathing problem, etc.
- ❖ Stressful situations like divorce, separation, death in the family, exams, unemployment, relationships issues.
- ❖ Withdrawal from a drug, alcohol, or medication
- ❖ Acute medical illness or hospitalization

Causes of Chronic or long term Insomnia : Majority of causes related to long term insomnia are either medical (physiologic) or psychological.

- ❖ **Physiologic Causes:**
  Causes such as disturbance in sleep wake balance, biological clock imbalance, or medical conditions like night Asthma, sleep apnea, acidity, degenerative diseases such as Alzheimer or Parkinson's, heart diseases, etc. are some of the physiological causes that may cause insomnia.

❖ **Psychological Causes:**

In a large number of cases, insomnia is an indicator of depression, acute stress, anxiety, and depression are the most common causes of sleeplessness. Stress could be emotional, mental, or physical. Apart from that extreme mood swings also termed as bipolar disorder, hormonal imbalances, and other mental health disorders like schizophrenia or split personality disorder are also some of the psychological causes of insomnia.

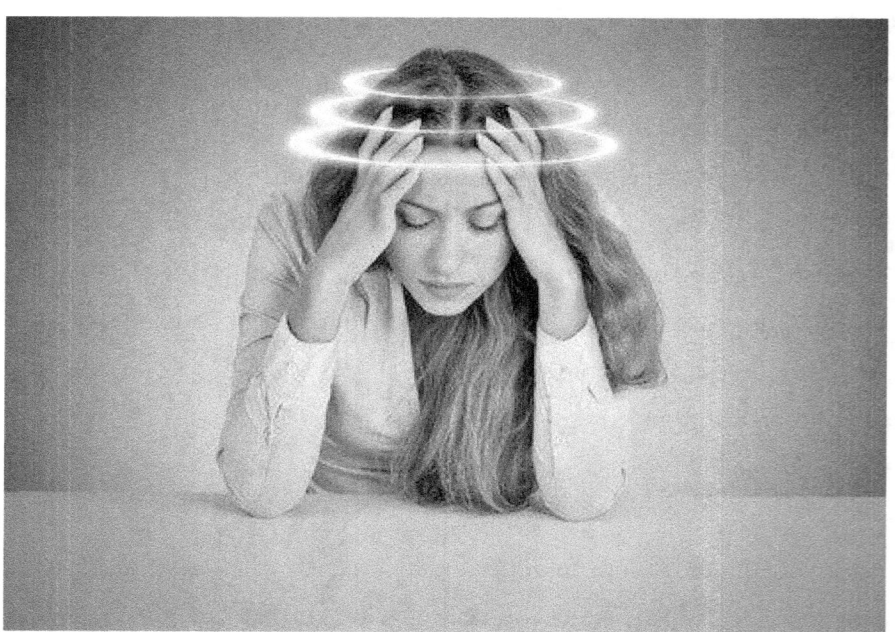

Other Causes of Insomnia:

❖ Pregnancy
❖ Hormonal shift during menstruation
❖ Genetic Conditions
❖ Sleeping next to a snoring partner
❖ Parasites

- ❖ Presence of Media Technology (TV, computer, video games, DVD player, mobile phone)
- ❖ More intake of caffeine and nicotine
- ❖ Increased intake of alcohol, can results in a disturbed night sleep.

Chapter #3: Signs and Symptoms

Common signs and symptoms of Insomnia are:

- ❖ Difficulty falling asleep at night
- ❖ Feeling tired after a night's sleep
- ❖ Sleepiness and fatigue during the daytime
- ❖ Waking up during the night
- ❖ Awakening early
- ❖ Irritability, anxiety, or depression
- ❖ Headaches
- ❖ Facing difficulty or no socializing
- ❖ Increase in errors related to coordination during the daytime
- ❖ Low concentration or focus
- ❖ Accidents because of fatigue
- ❖ Difficulty remembering things
- ❖ Lack of energy
- ❖ Fatigue

Insomnia is usually related to other problem. Insomnia without a cause related to any other problem is very rare. These problems could be:

- ❖ **Stress:** The stress levels may vary from minor professional and personal stress to severe stress like a separation, divorce, death, unemployment, etc.
- ❖ **Sleep Disorders:** There are some sleep disorders that may cause insomnia or worsen an already existing insomnia condition. For example, people with restless leg syndrome (creeping sensation in the

leg caused during sleep which are relieved with regular leg movement) may face a tough time falling asleep

- ❖ **Medication:** Insomnia may also be caused by or may be a side effect of a prescribed or over the counter medication. For example, many common cold or allergy medications contain pseudoephedrine which may cause difficulty in falling asleep. Other anti depressants and drugs used to treat high blood pressure, ADHD, etc may also cause insomnia.
- ❖ **Medical Condition:** People who have restricted mobility due to a physical illness or who experience pain and discomfort due to a medical problem may face difficulty in falling or staying asleep throughout the night. Insomnia caused due to medical conditions is most common in older adults.
- ❖ **Pregnancy:** Insomnia during pregnancy, particularly third trimester, is very common when the baby is growing rapidly putting pressure on the uterus.

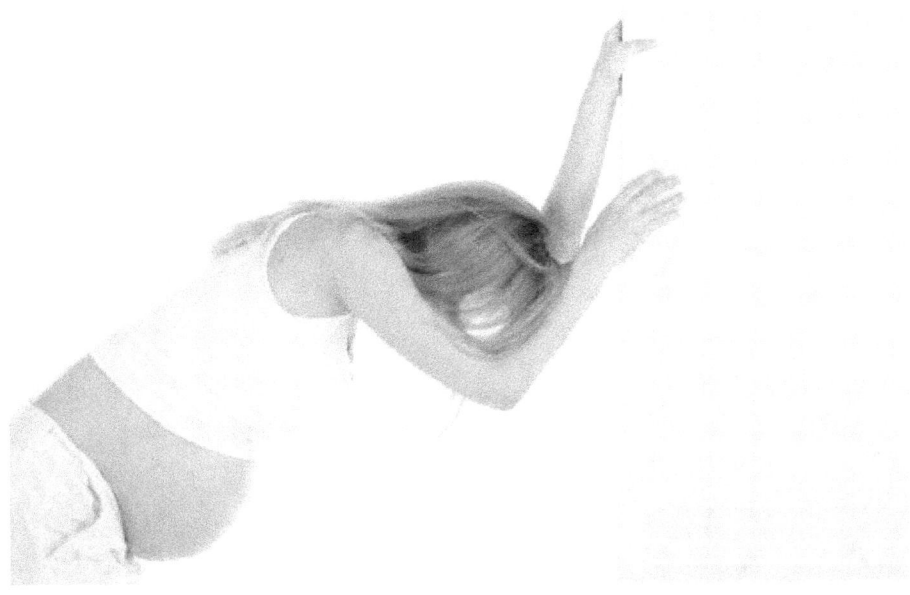

- ❖ **Age:** As people age, they tend to have more chronic health problems which may result in insomnia.
- ❖ **Heat flashes and Menopause:** Hormonal changes and heat flashes caused due to menopause may also result into insomnia.
- ❖ **Lifestyle:** Irregular eating and sleeping schedules may also result in insomnia.
- ❖ **Consumption of alcohol:** Alcohol intake before bedtime may cause frequent awakening resulting in disturbed sleep throughout the night.
- ❖ **Caffeine and nicotine:** Both caffeine and nicotine prevent you from falling asleep.
- ❖ **Allergens:** Some people are allergic to some foods and if consumed, it may result in insomnia or disrupted sleep.
- ❖ **Environment:** The environment where one sleeps may also cause insomnia. Factors like light, noise, and extreme temperatures, may interfere with the sleep.

Tests and Treatments

Chapter #4: Tests to diagnose Insomnia

Self Test:

If you feel that you are suffering from insomnia, ask yourself the following questions:

- Does it take more than 30 minutes for you to fall asleep?
- Do you wake up in the night and face trouble returning to sleep?
- Do you have daytime fatigue, low energy levels, sleepiness, or mood swings during the day?
- Do you give yourself time to get enough sleep (for 6-8 hours)?
- Do you have a quiet, dark bedroom environment?
- Do you keep your electronics (TV, cell phone, tab) in silent mode or out of your bedroom?

If your answer to all the above questions is 'yes', then you have insomnia. If this sleep condition is new and it has only been a few weeks, try to self help by following a good sleep routine. If your problem has continued for more than two to three months, you might want to consult a physician or your family doctor. They may further refer you to a board certified sleep physician.

Before your appointment to a board certified sleep physician, your doctor may ask you to keep a sleep diary for a couple of weeks just to learn about your sleep patterns and what exactly the reason behind your insomnia is.

In your sleep diary, you may want to record the time when you go to sleep, time when you wake up, along with how many times you woke up, and for how long you were awake at night. This sleep diary not only gives clues about your sleep habits and what is causing you insomnia but will also help your doctor to suggest a treatment course for you.

A board certified sleep physician will diagnose your insomnia and work with his team to treat it. He will ask questions related to your medical history, any medications which you might be taking including over the counter drugs.

To start with, you may have a detailed question answer sessions with the sleep therapist related to your personal and professional lives. These sessions are just to know more about what exactly is the stress that is causing the bigger problem.

You may be given a written questionnaire to know about your mental and emotional well being. A blood test may also be recommended if the specialist feels that there is an underlying medical problem that is causing insomnia.

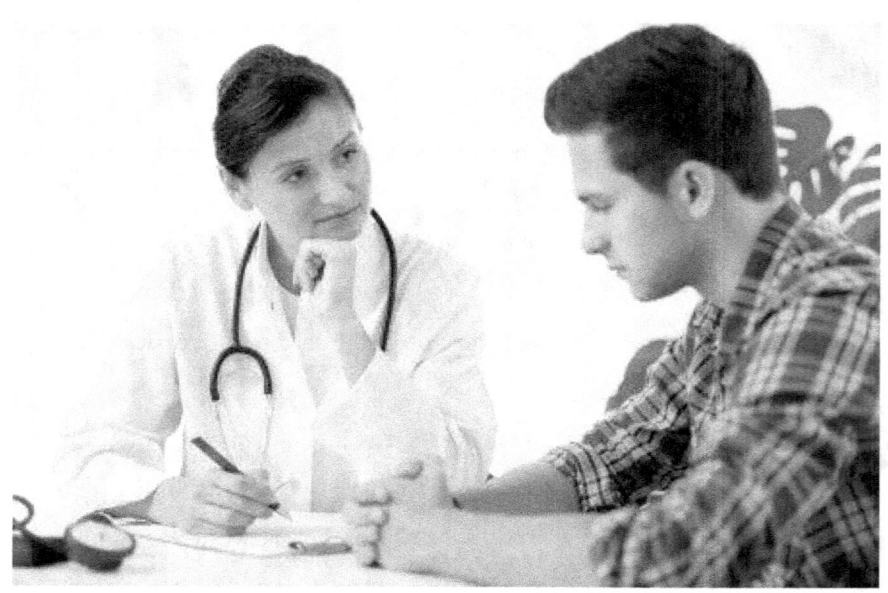

Physicians may screen for psychiatric disorders, drug and alcohol use etc. One may need an overnight sleep study, if the sleep specialist suspects a sleeping disorder or sleep apnea.

Other tests which may be conducted are:

- **Polysomnograph:** It is an overnight sleeping test that records sleep patterns.
- **Actigraphy:** In this a small wrist device is given called an actigraph that measures movement and sleep wake patterns.

Chapter #5: Treatment Options

Most types of insomnia get resolved, when the underlying cause is removed. Thus, treatment for insomnia majorly focuses on understanding the underlying cause of sleeping problem. Once identified, the cause can be treated or corrected properly. In addition to the main cause treatment, treatments such as behavioral and medical both can be applied as complimenting therapies.

In case of chronic insomnia, a board certified sleep physician, may recommend a combination of treatment such as:

- **Practice sleep hygiene:** Sleep hygiene is a set bedtime routine which you can do every night before hitting the bed to improve your sleep. You can also improve your sleep hygiene by not over doing or under sleeping, by exercising daily, by avoiding caffeine and nicotine, by making your bedroom environment comfortable and by using relaxation techniques like meditation and muscle relaxation.

- **Cognitive Behavioral Therapy:** Cognitive Behavioral Therapy for Insomnia or CBTi refers to the thoughts and behaviors that keep you away from having a sound sleep. CBTi helps you learn new strategies and techniques such as stress reduction, sleep schedule management, relaxation, etc. There are trained specialists who provide CBTi therapies.

- **Stimulus Control Therapy:** It consists of few simple steps that are useful for patients with chronic insomnia. These are:
  - Go to bed only when sleepy.
  - Avoid napping during daytime

- o If you are not able to sleep for 30 minutes in bed, it's better to wake up and try relaxation techniques
- o No TV watching, eating, reading in bed. Use your bed only for sleeping and sexual activities.
- o Do not oversleep. Set your alarm clock to get up at a fixed time each morning.
- **Medication:** The board certified specialist may prescribe a medication to treat insomnia. There are sleeping pills which are specifically approved to treat insomnia. These are known as hypnotics. Overtime, you may build a tolerance to these medications. There are also some medicines that treat other problems but may also help in insomnia. It is purely on your doctor's description as to which medicines will suit you and how the medical treatment for the same should be continued. Remember, these medications should always be taken under the prescription of a medical practitioner.

  The course of the medication may change as your medical condition improves. Your sleep specialist may also change some of the medications that you may be taking currently, if he suspects that those drugs may be responsible for insomnia.

Recovery from insomnia:

Recovering from insomnia may vary depending upon the cause:

- If the insomnia is caused by a jet lag, its symptoms may clear up in a few days.
- If you are depressed and have anxiety for many months, it's unlikely that the symptoms may disappear by themselves. You may require an expert's advice and treatment.

- Recovery will also depend on your medical conditions such as heart failure, chronic pain, various syndromes, etc.

Chapter #6: Natural Remedies for Treating Insomnia: Foods, Supplements, and Herbs

Though there is always an option of trying prescribed sleeping aids, but there are several natural remedies for insomnia too. Lifestyle changes, certain foods, supplements, and herbs can also help in getting a restful sleep.

❖ **Sleep time snacks:** Experts suggest that there are people who need something to binge upon to get a good night sleep. A combination of carbohydrate and protein works wonders as a sleep inducing snack. For example: half a banana with a tablespoon of peanut butter or a whole wheat cracker with some cheese. You may eat one of these snacks around 30 minutes before hitting the bed.

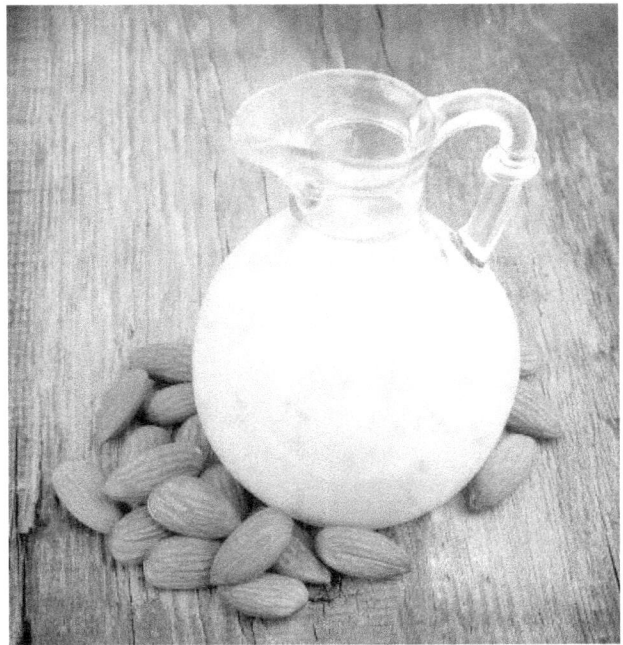

❖ **Warm milk:** Warm milk on the other hand is grandmother's remedy for a good night sleep. Sipping warm milk before bed time helps the brain to make melatonin (our body's internal pacemaker that controls our timing and drive for sleep). Almond milk is an excellent source of calcium. Plus, sipping over warm milk soothes you and helps you to fall asleep soon.

Apart from the regular medications, there are also some very popular **herbal medicines** available. But it's recommended to take any of the medicines as per a medical practitioner's prescription.

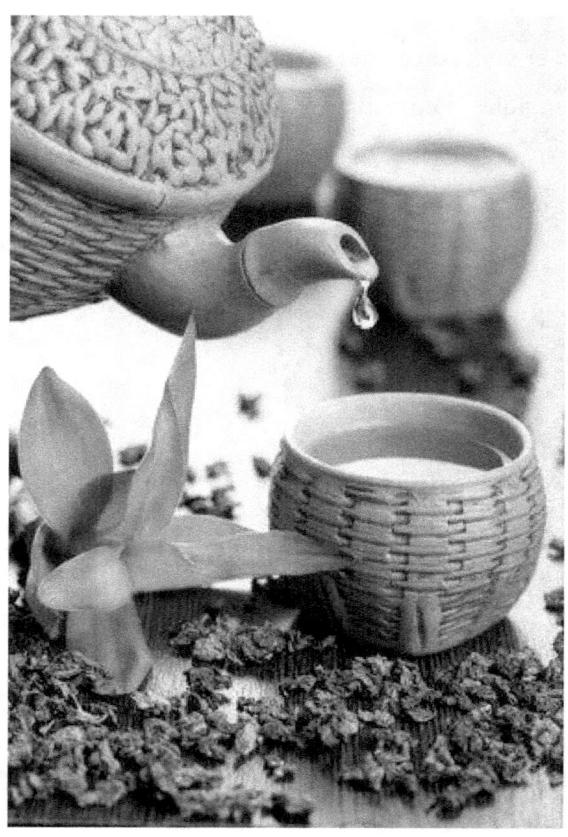

The following are some of the herbal medicines:

- **Valerian root:** It is a popular herbal medication especially in the United States and has shown good results in some patients with chronic insomnia. This medicinal herb has been used to treat sleep problems since ancient times. If you try valerian, you need to be patient as it may take around a couple of weeks to show its effect. It's better to talk to your doctor before taking it.

- **Chamomile:** Though it gives a relaxing effect to body and mind but it has not shown any real benefit in treating insomnia. Similarly St. Johns Wort is also a very popular herbal medication with less of real benefits in the treatment of insomnia.

- **Lavender:** Lavender oil may encourage sleep in some people dealing with insomnia as it is very calming. Taking a hot water bath with lavender oil before bedtime will help in relaxing body and mind.

Other herbal or natural sleeping aids such as kava kava, dogwood, and L-tryptophan are said to be associated with potential side effects when used for treating insomnia.

- ❖ **Magnesium:** Research shows that Magnesium plays a vital role in inducing sleep. Even a marginal deficiency of it may prevent the brain from settling down at night. So consuming foods that are rich in magnesium may also help in inducing sleep. Examples of foods having high magnesium content are: Almonds, pumpkin seeds, green leafy vegetables, wheat germ, etc. If opting for taking magnesium supplements, it's recommended to consult your doctor as Magnesium may interact with other medications and excess of it may even cause serious health issues.

❖ **L-theanine:** L-theanine is an amino acid which is found in green tea leaves. It helps in fighting stress and anxiety that interferes with a sound sleep. It increases the feel good hormone in our body and reduces heart rate and immune responses to stress. Thus inducing relaxing waves in the brain. Be sure to take your doctor's recommended dose.

Self Help

Chapter #7: Tips for controlling Insomnia

It's not quantity, but the quality of sleep one gets at night that makes the waking hours more fresh and energetic. How we feel during the daytime depends a lot on how we slept last night.

One can easily cure the daytime fatigue and sleepiness by adopting few tips in their sleeping schedule.

The following tips will help you to have a sound sleep and be energetic, mentally alert, more productive, and emotionally balanced throughout the day.

Tip 1: Set a sleep schedule

Be consistent in your bed time routine. Set a sleep schedule (i.e going to bed and waking up at a particular time every day). Setting this schedule is one of the easiest and important strategy to wake up feeling more refreshed and energized.

Sleeping the same number of hours at different times of the day will not work. What matters is consistency.

This consistency of sleep-wake schedule will help in setting up your body's internal clock. It's better to set a realistic bed time that works with your lifestyle. Set a time when you naturally feel tired. When you get good night sleep, you wake up naturally without an alarm. But if you require an alarm to wake you up, you may need to go to bed a bit early.

Tip 2: Avoid sleeping late on weekends

Though it may be tempting to sleep a couple of hours more on weekends but remember a couple of hours difference may upset your internal body clock. The more difference between weekday/weekend bedtimes, the more you will experience the jetlag type symptoms. In case, you sleep late on a particular night, try to opt for a daytime nap instead of a late wake up morning. This will help in keeping your sleep wake rhythm intact thus reducing the chances of insomnia.

Tip 3: Avoid Napping

Though napping seems to be a good option for instant recharge of the body and making up for the lost sleep hours, but if you are suffering from insomnia, it's better to avoid napping during the daytime or restricting the time limit to 15 to 20 minutes during early afternoon hours.

Tip 4: Avoid after meal drowsiness

If you feel drowsy after meals especially after dinner, try to get off your couch and indulge yourself in chores like washing dishes, calling someone, cleaning, etc. forgetting sleep. If you give in to the drowsiness, you may wake up in the middle of the night and may face trouble getting back to sleep.

Tip 5: Control light in your bedroom

A natural hormone called melatonin is controlled by exposure to light and helps in regulating sleep-wake cycle. Our brain secretes more melatonin when it is dark, thus making us feel sleepy and when its light, melatonin secretion is less thus making us more alert.

Now with modern lifestyle, our body's natural production of this hormone has been altered. Spending long hours away from natural light inside our rooms with bright lights from LED's, TV's, Computer screens, etc, can make our brain think that it's time to wake up. Thus, shifting our sleep wake cycle and impacting our daytime wakefulness and making our brain sleepy.

Since we cannot avoid the modern day technology, you may want to follow certain pointers to keep your hormone, as well as, your sleep wake cycle in check:

During the day:

Spend more time in the sunlight by either eating your breakfast by a sunny window, exercising, having your morning tea in balcony, taking work breaks in day light, avoiding sun glasses. This way the light on your face will make you feel alert.

At night:

Try to limit exposure to blue light emitted by electronics like phone, tablet, computer, TV screens, etc as these can be disruptive and may interfere with your sleep. If need be, try to turn down the brightness, if you prefer listening to music or audio books.

At bedtime, ensure there is no device that emits light. The darker the room, the easier it is to fall asleep. Try using heavy curtains or window shades to block any outside light. In case, you wake up in the midst of night, try not to turn on the lights or if you need, try turning on a foot lamp of dim light or use a small flash light. This will make it easier for you to fall back to sleep soon.

Tip 6: Smart eating and drinking

What you put in your body plays an important role in how well you sleep. It's very important to watch what you eat for your dinner and in the hours leading to your bedtime. Try to stay away from big meals at night. If feasible shift your dinner time to earlier in the evening. Keeping your dinner light and staying away from foods that take long to get digested like fried, fatty foods can keep sleep problems at bay.

Cut down on your caffeine and alcohol intake. Also be careful about spicy or acidic foods at dinner since they may cause heartburn or stomach problems.

For some, night time snacking may help in sleeping better and for others, eating before bed may lead to indigestion resulting into disturbed sleep. It's better to experiment and determine what suits you and what your optimum evening meal is and snack routine.

Though anything light may be a good idea as a bedtime snack, you may try having a small bowl of low sugar cereal with milk, a bowl of yogurt, half a sandwich, or a banana.

Tip 7: Exercise regularly

Regular exercise not only helps you sleep better by increasing the time you spend in deep sleep but also helps to decrease symptoms of insomnia and sleep apnea.

Even walking for 10-15 minutes a day can do wonders to your sleep quality. This tip will not work over night, regularly exercising for a few months, will gradually improve your sleep, so it's better to focus on building an exercise habit that stays and your sleep quality is sure to improve.

A few items to remember when exercising, it will increase your metabolism, your body temperature, and active the hormone cortisol. These are all great things, but if exercise occurs too close to bedtime, it may hinder your sleep. Try to avoid doing any exercise at least 3 hours before bedtime. Some people find they need up to 6 hours to cool completely down from a workout, so you will have to test yourself. Also, indulging in light stretching and relaxing exercises, like yoga, as part of your bedtime routine, will help in promoting sleep.

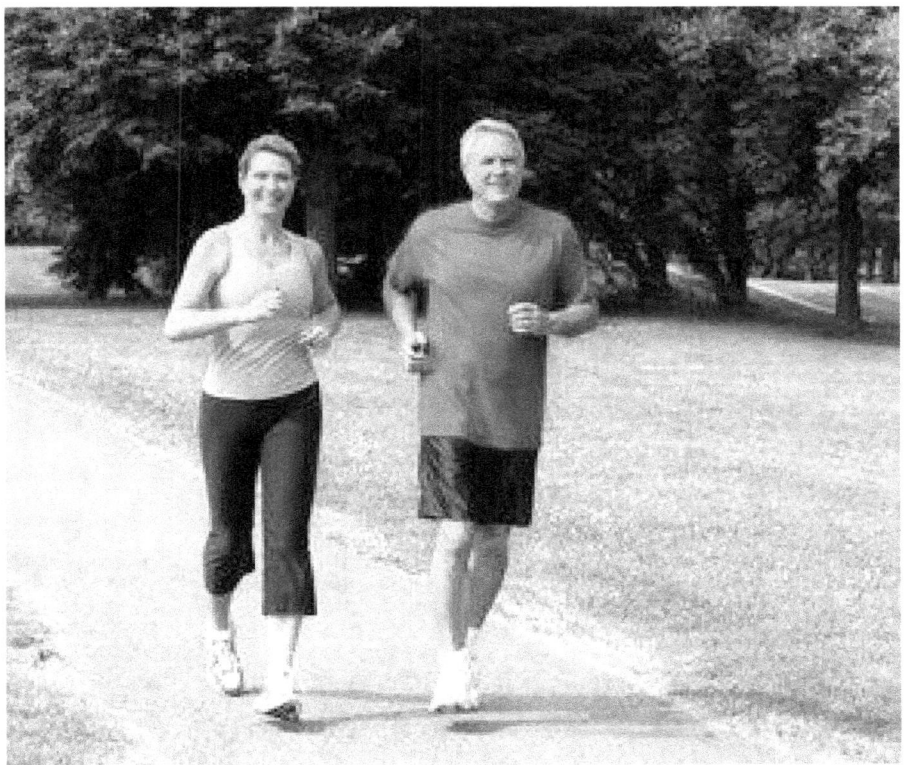

Tip 8: Make a bedtime routine

A peaceful bedtime routine gives signals to your brain to let go of the stress and unwind. Routine such as:

- Taking a warm water bath
- Doing a little bit of stretching
- Listening to soft soothing music
- Reading a book or a magazine

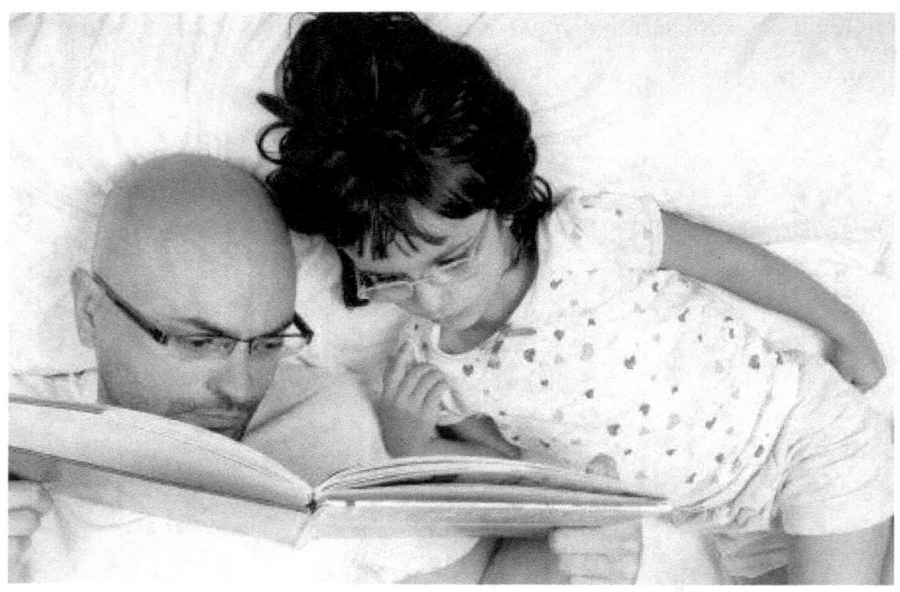

You may also wind down by indulging in your favorite hobby or by making preparations for the next day. Remember to dim the lights as you wind down.

Chapter #8: Relaxation Techniques for better sleep

If you seem to be excessively worrying, thus keeping your mind active and awake, you need to learn about managing your thoughts and relaxing yourself before you hit the bed. If the thoughts linger around in your mind, they will not only disturb your night's sleep but will also spoil your next day.

In this fast pace world, we all work under pressure. Stress could be from work, school, family, etc. If any of the stress is keeping you awake at night, you may need to learn how to control this stress and channel it in a calm way.

Practicing some of the relaxation techniques before bedtime is a great way to calm your body and mind and prepare for sleep.

Following are some of the relaxation techniques for better sleep:

1. **Deep Breathing:** Lie down on your bed, close your eyes and take slow deep breaths. Make each breath deeper than the last one.
2. **Visualize a calm place:** Lie down on your bed, close your eyes, and visualize a peaceful, restful, place. Concentrate on how relaxing it feels.
3. **Muscle Relaxation:** Start with your toes. Tense all the muscles tightly and then release the tension completely. Release the tension on each and every muscle of your body starting from toes to forehead.

While performing any of the relaxing techniques, keep your room dark, quiet, and cool. Try to keep noise to the minimal.

Also ensure that your bed is comfortable. Use good comfortable pillows or neck rest so that you do not get an aching back or neck once you wake up.

Try different levels of mattress firmness, foam, softness, elasticity, etc. Use pillows wherever you need support.

It's better to reserve your bedroom for sleeping and relaxing. If you relate your bedroom with work or other activities, it will be difficult to relax and unwind at night.

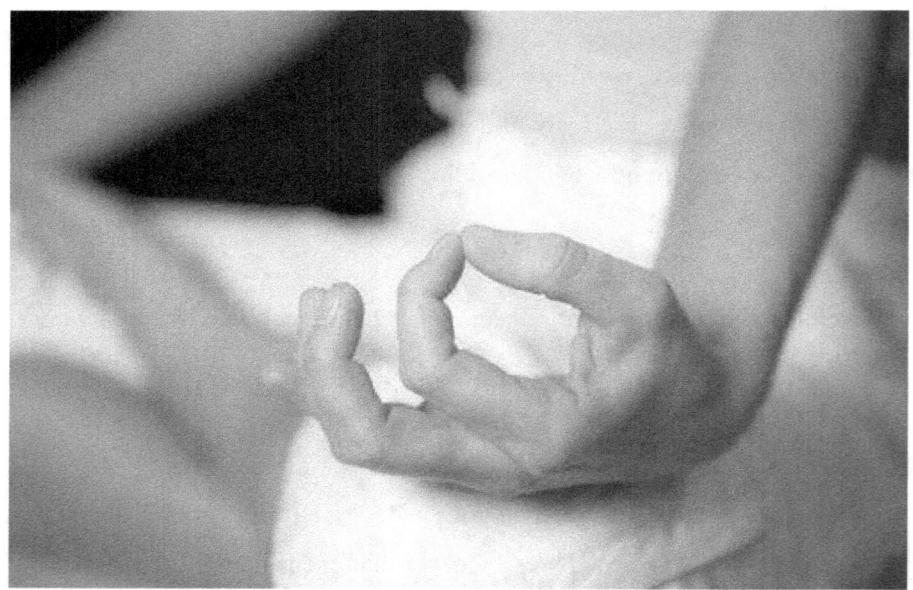

Chapter #9: Ways to get back to sleep

It's pretty normal to wake up for a short while at night. A good sleeper may not even remember this and get back to sleep fast. But in case, you wake up at night and find it difficult to fall back to sleep, following tips may help :

1. **Do not think about getting back to sleep:** The very worry of not able to sleep again hinders with the sleep. It's better to keep your body in a relaxed position. Does not stress too much as it will keep you awake for an even longer period.

2. **Practice relaxing technique :** Do deep breathing and relax your body. You may even think or say the word 'Ahhhh' with each breath.

3. **Make relaxation your goal and not sleep :** Even though you find it hard to get back to sleep, do not move out of your bed and try to relax yourself. Although relaxation is not a replacement for sleep but try to remind yourself that rest and relaxing will help in rejuvenating the body for the next day.

4. **Indulge in a quiet, non stimulating activity:** If you have been awake for more than 20-25 minutes and there seems to be no sign of getting back to sleep, try engaging yourself in a quiet, non stimulating activity such as reading a book. Remember to keep the lights dim.

5. **Avoid screen time:** Once you wake up in the middle of the night, avoid looking at any of the screens such as TV, cell phones, computers, tablets, etc as these lights act as brain stimulators and will keep you awake for a longer period.

6. **Sip on a herbal tea:** Sipping over a cup of herbal team may help you feel relaxed and get back to sleep soon.

7. **Postpone your thoughts :** If you wake up at night feeling anxious or with a great idea, it's better to write it down on a piece of paper and fall back to sleep and postpone the thoughts to the other day when you are fresh and more productive and creative after a good night's rest.

Chapter #10: When to contact your doctor

If, in spite of your self help and efforts, still you are facing problems of insomnia as in:

- Regular day time fatigue and sleepiness
- Difficulty falling or staying asleep
- Morning headaches
- Inability to move while falling asleep or waking up
- Sizzling sensation in your arms or legs at night
- Pain or difficulty breathing at night may indicate emergency medical care.

If these symptoms last for three to four weeks, you may need medical help.

Your doctor may recommend you to a sleep disorder specialist or cognitive behavioral therapist if your insomnia:

- Has not responded to self help
- Is getting worse
- Is causing issues at work, home, or school
- Is resulting in symptoms like chest pain or shortness of breath.

Conclusion:

Insomnia is a common problem. In many cases, it is just for a temporary phase and gets treated once the underlying cause is identified. There are many people who find a treatment that works for them either with the self help techniques or with the help of a board certified sleep medicine physician.

In general, transient or temporary insomnia gets resolved when the underlying root cause or the trigger is corrected or removed. Most people only seek medical attention when their insomnia becomes chronic.

The main focus of an insomnia treatment is directed towards finding the cause. Once a root cause is identified, it is important to manage and control the underlying cause as this alone may eliminate the insomnia problem all together.

Treating just the symptoms of insomnia without understanding and addressing the main cause is rarely successful. In majority of cases, chronic insomnia gets cured if it is properly evaluated for both medical and psychiatric causes.

Studies have clearly shown that a combination of medical as well as psychiatric treatments is more successful in treating insomnia than any one alone.

Here's to wishing you a quality night sleep.

About the Author

Dr. Usman is an MD, now pursuing his post-graduation degree. As a medical doctor, he has deep insight in all aspects of health, fitness and nutrition.

He is a certified nutritionist and a personal trainer. With these qualifications, he has helped countless people reach their health, fitness and weight loss goals.

Dr. Usman is an avid researcher with 20+ publications in internationally accepted peer reviewed journals.

He is an accomplished writer with more than 5 years of writing experience. In this time, he has produced countless blogs, articles and research work on topics related to health, fitness and nutrition.

He is a published author with more than 100+ books published and several more in the pipe line.

Finally, he runs his own blog and posts health, fitness and nutrition related articles there regularly. You can visit his blog at http://hcures.com/.

Check out some of the other JD-Biz Publishing books

Gardening Series on Amazon

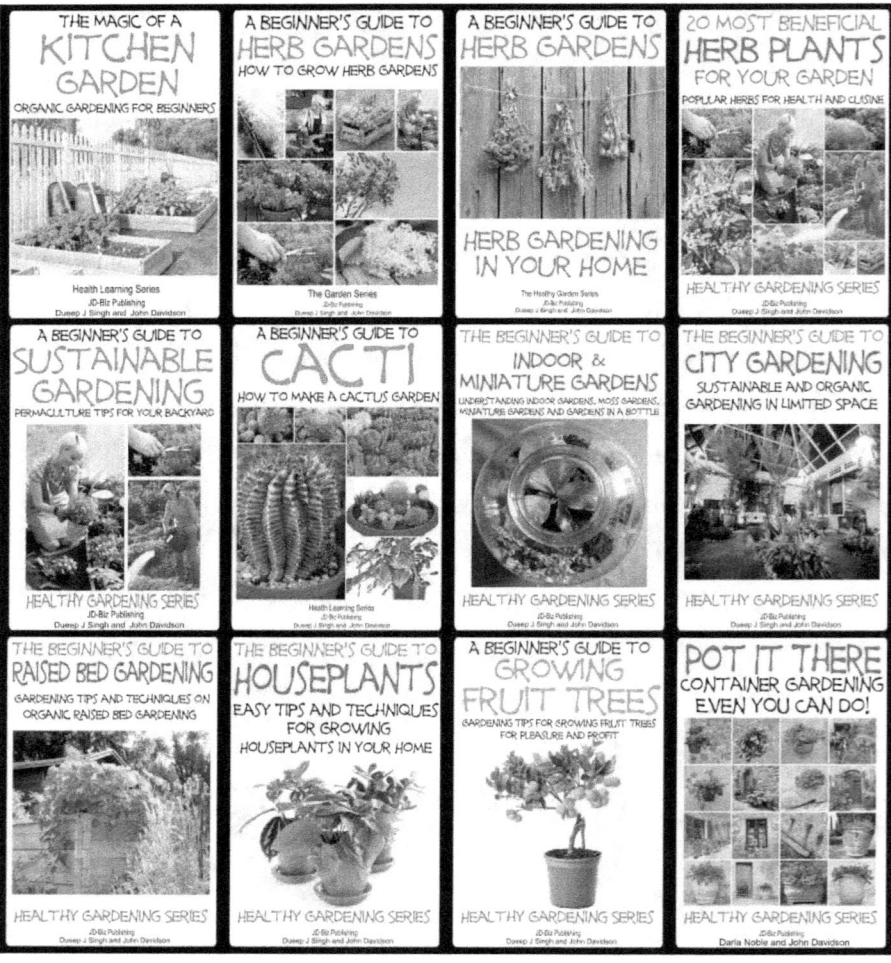

Download Free Books!
http://MendonCottageBooks.com

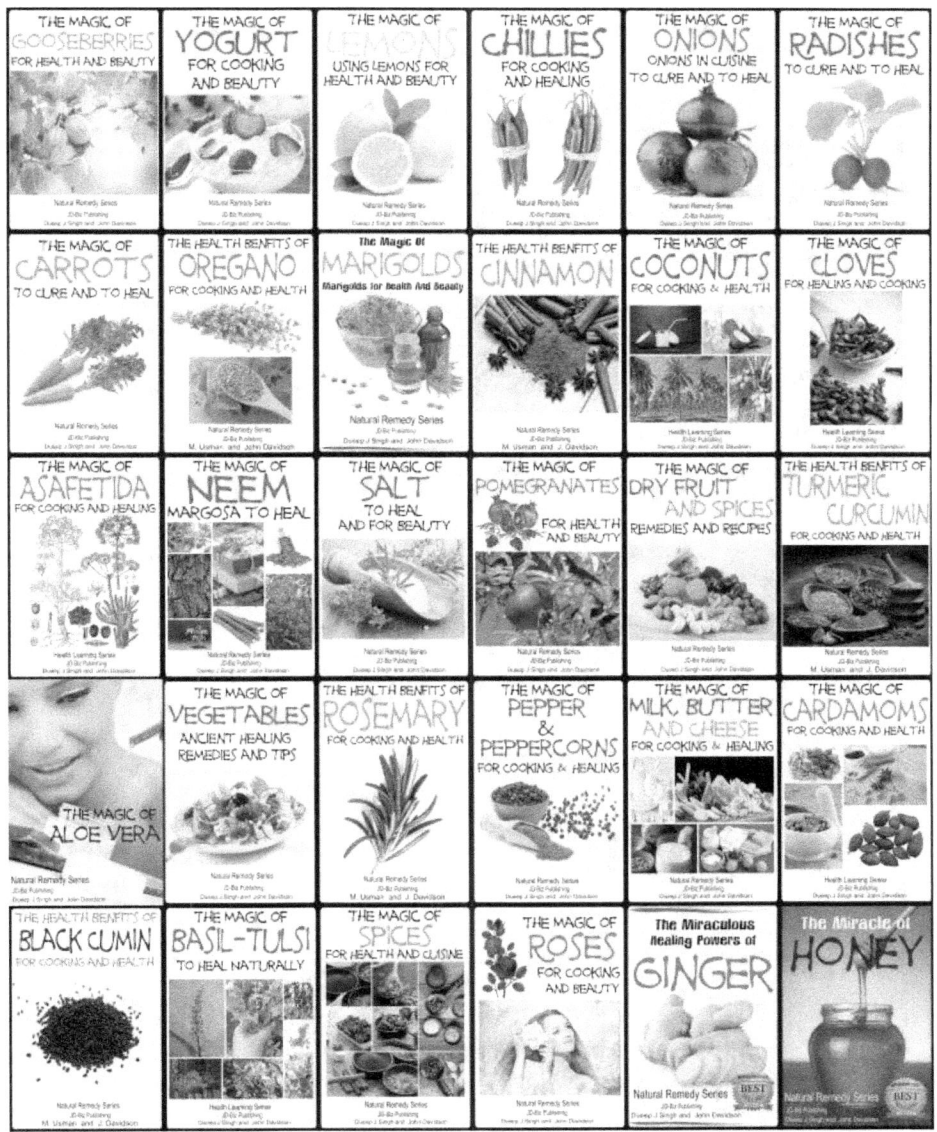

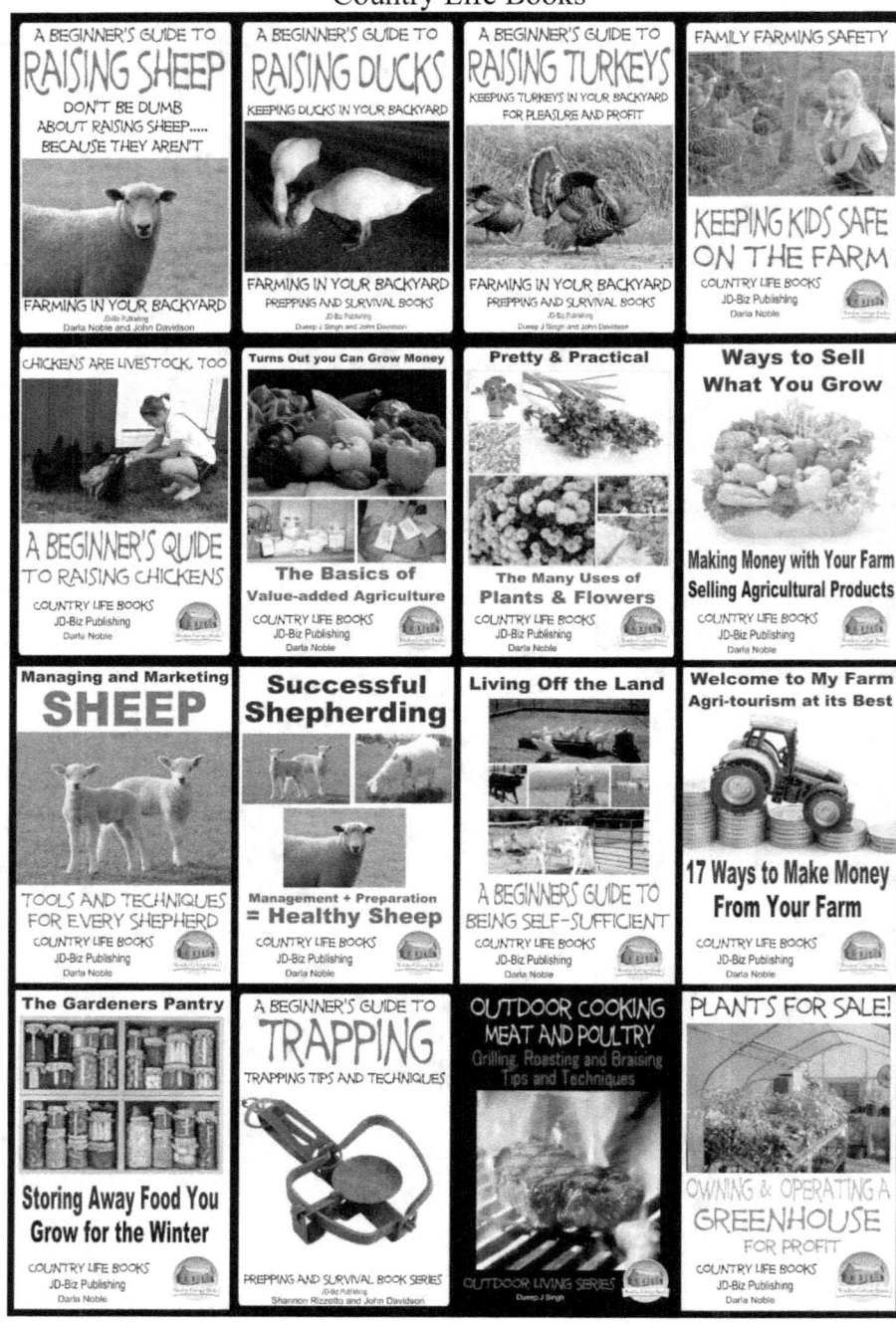

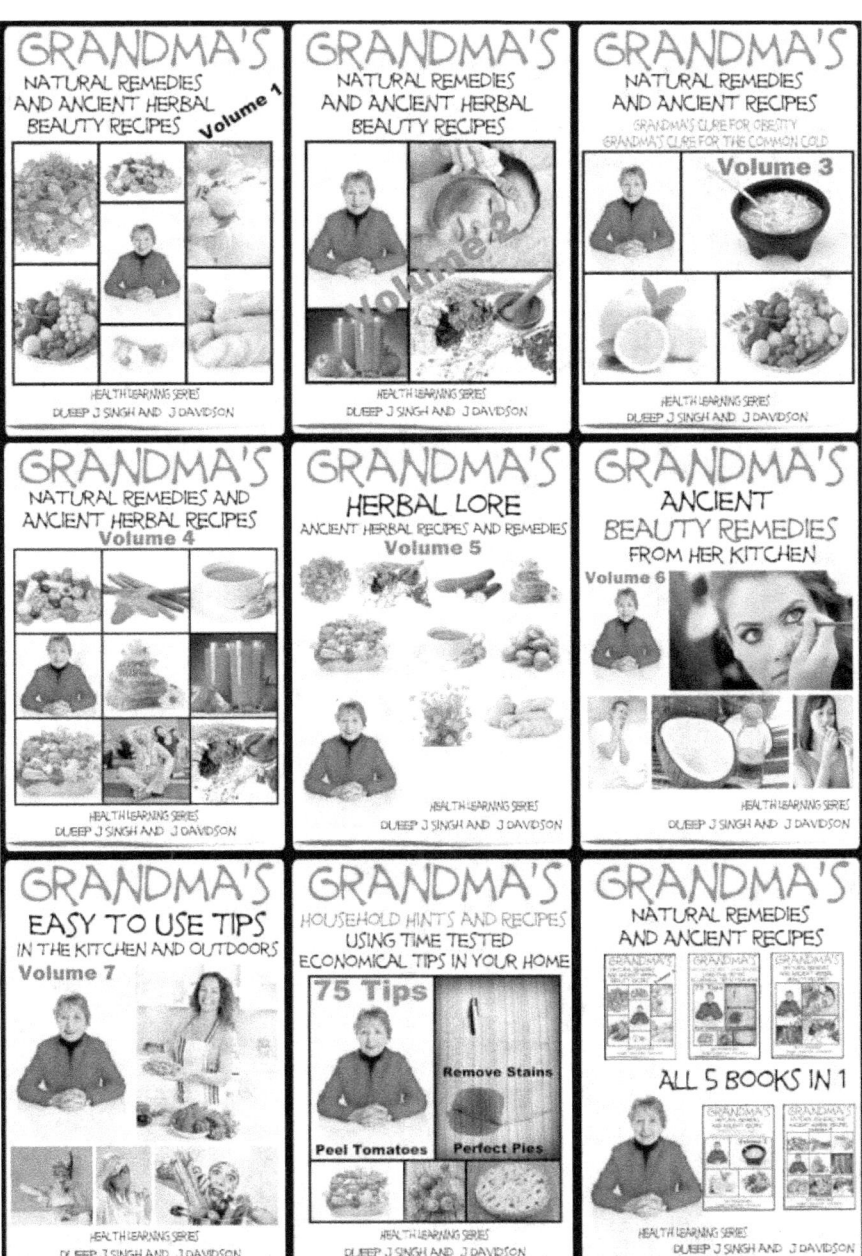

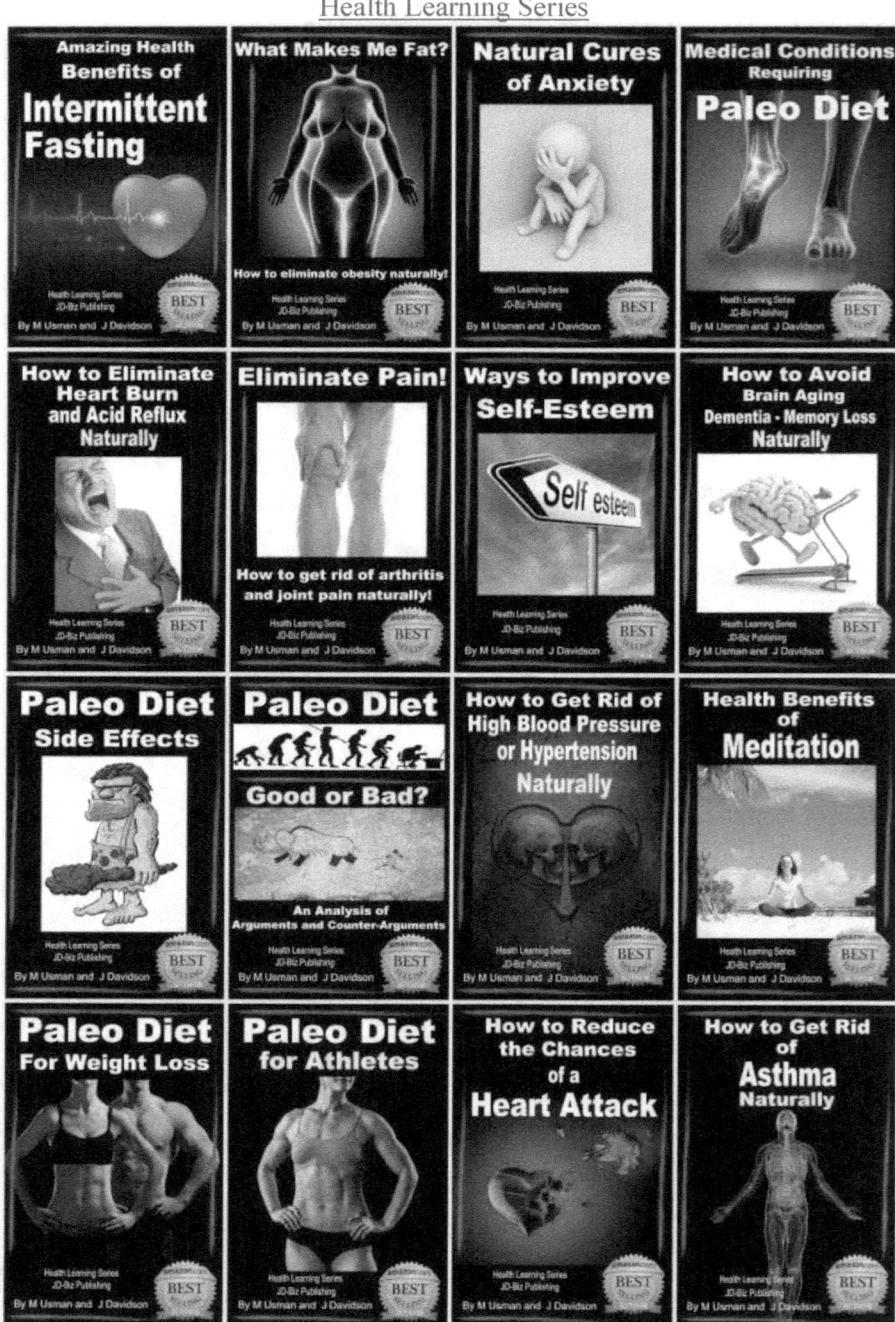

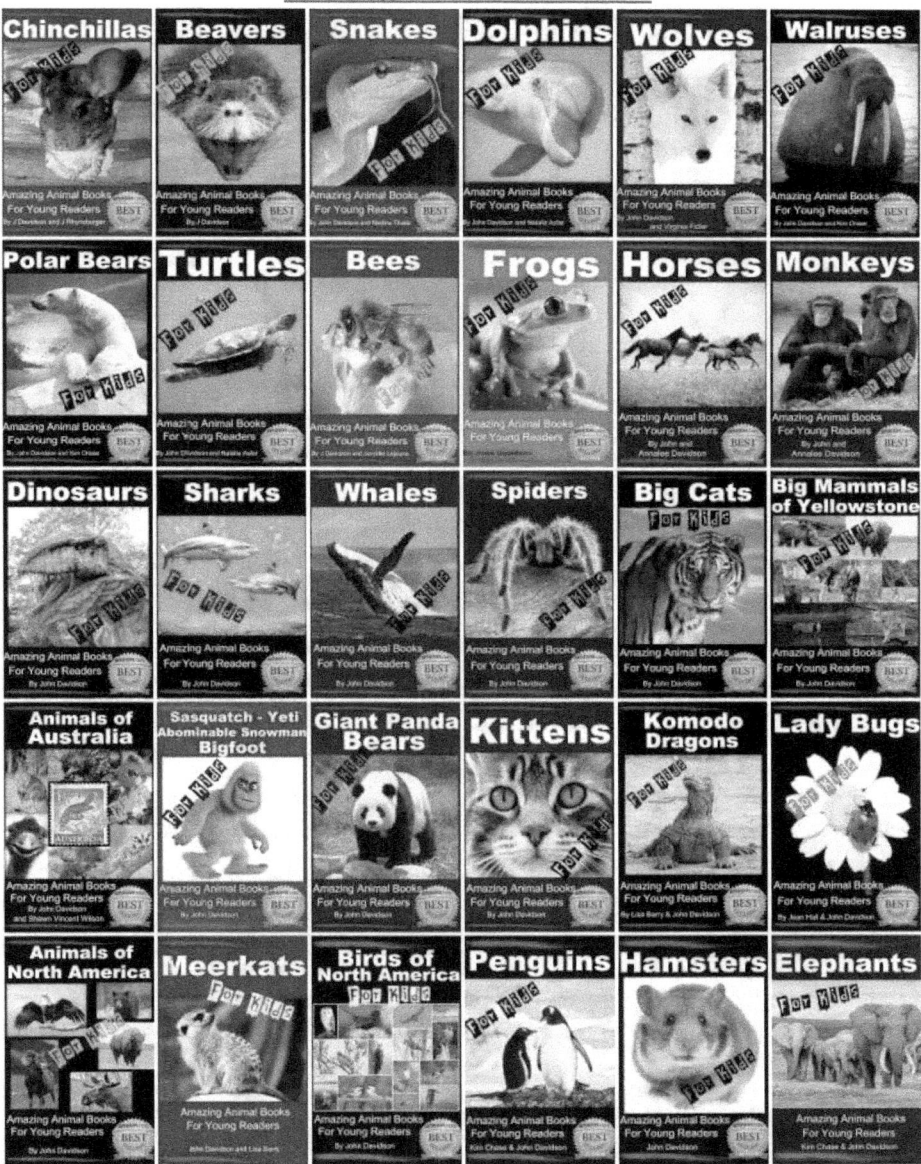

Learn To Draw Series

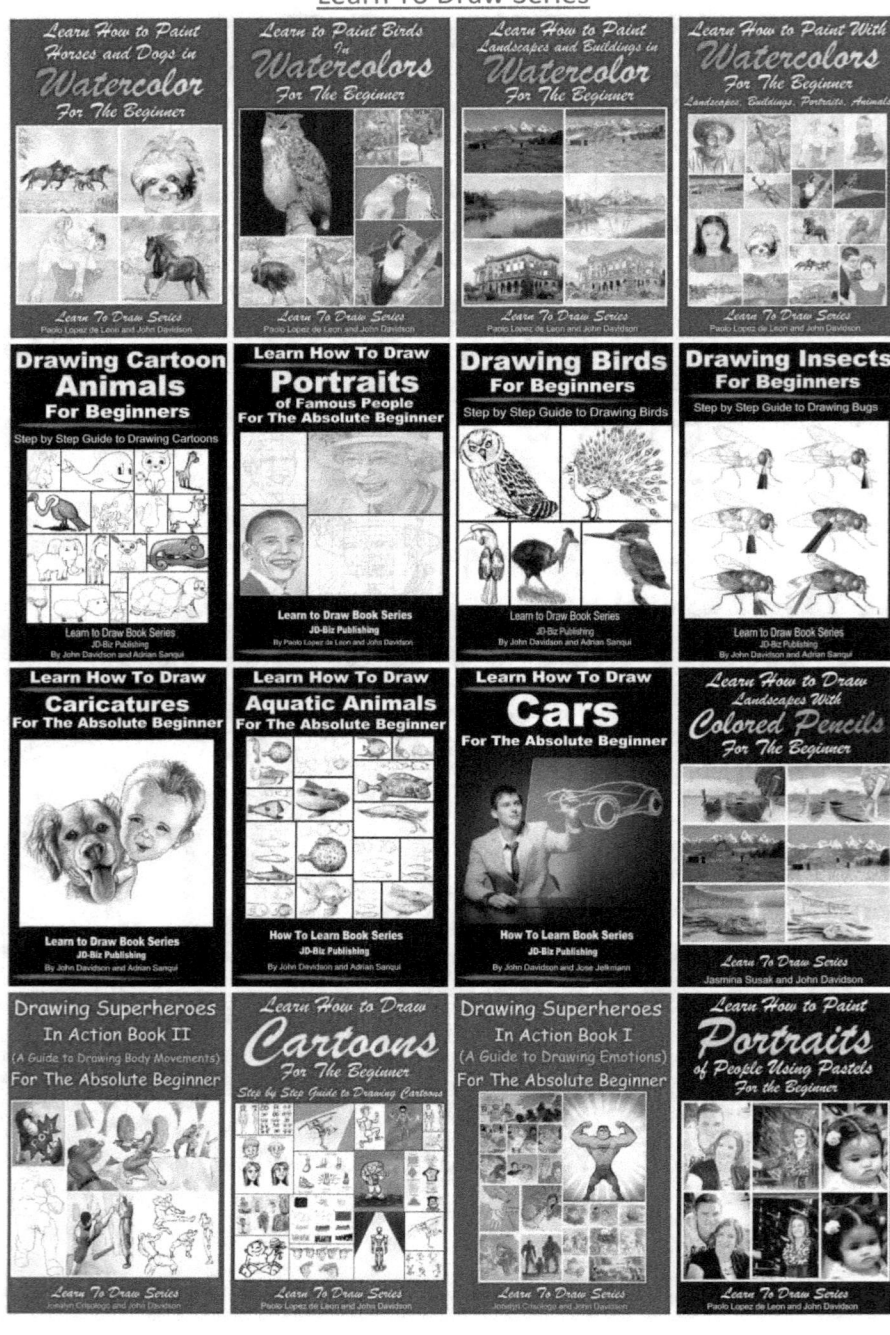

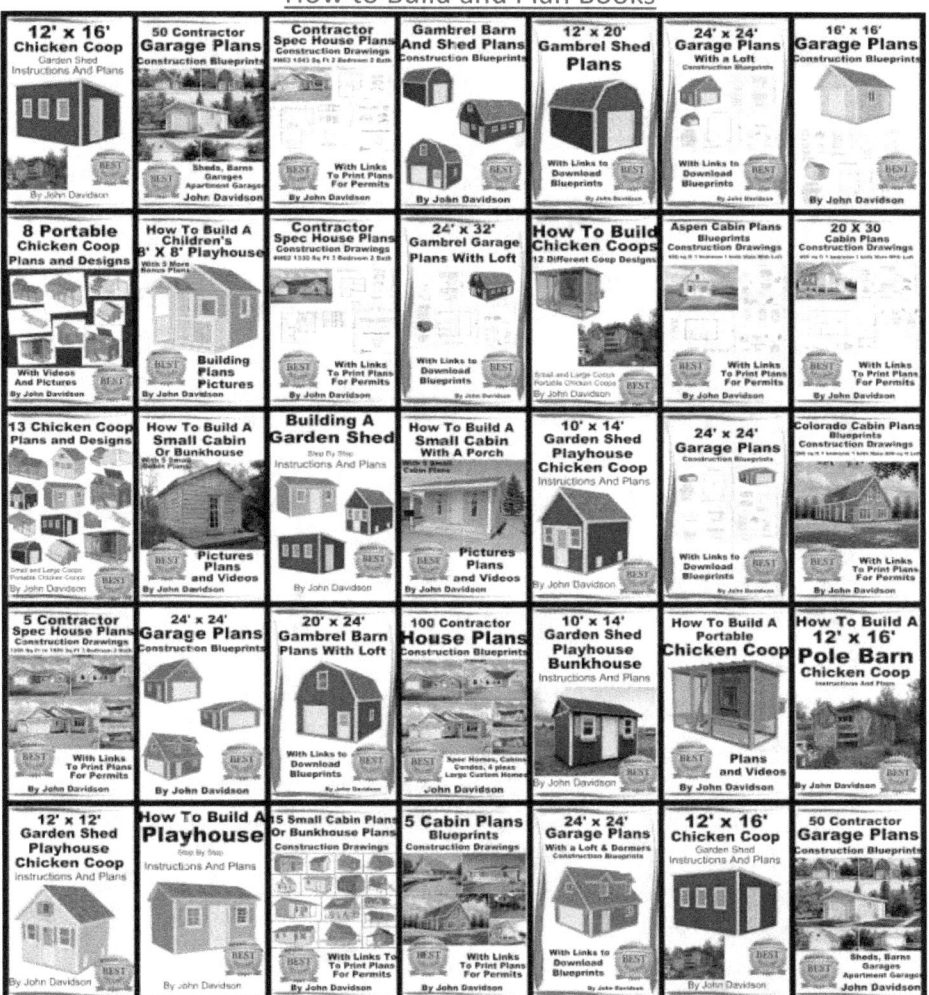

Entrepreneur Book Series

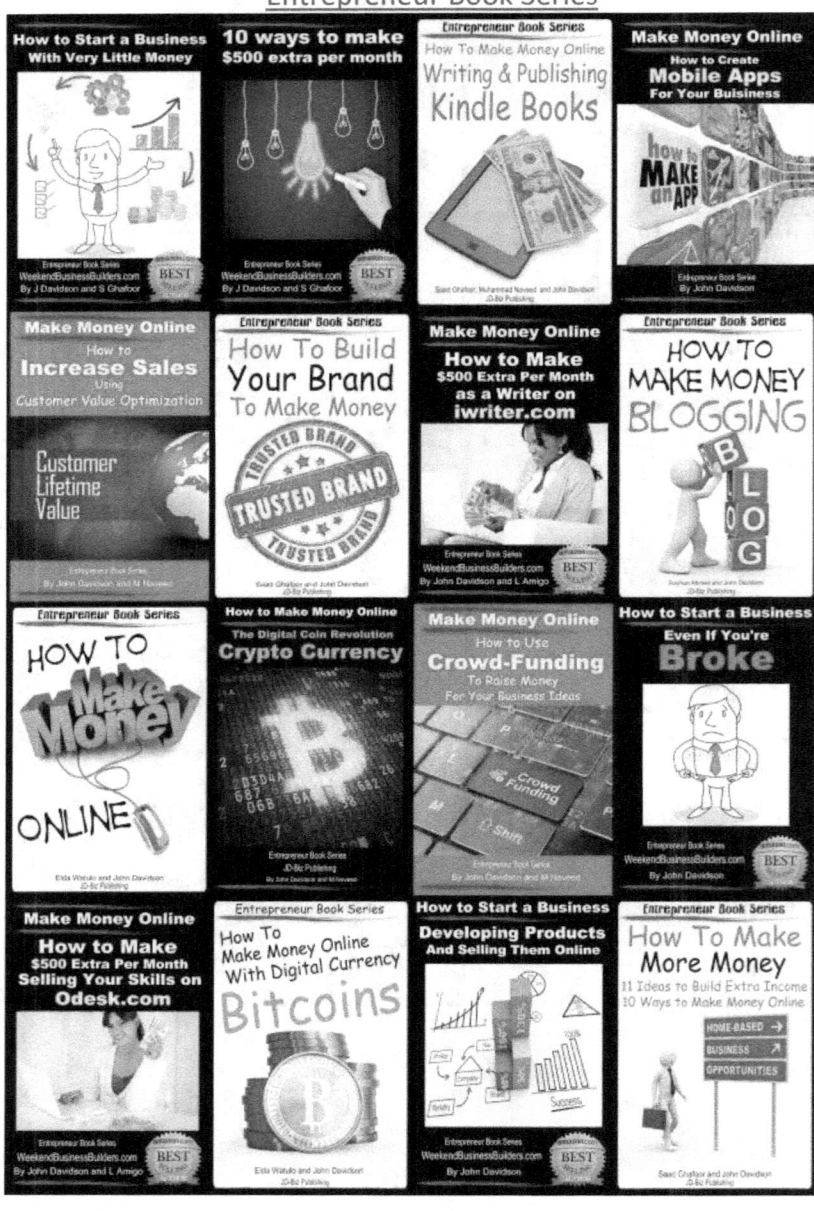

Our books are available at

1. Amazon.com

2. Barnes and Noble

3. Itunes

4. Kobo

5. Smashwords

6. Google Play Books

Publisher

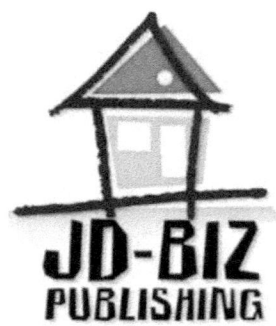

JD-Biz Corp

P O Box 374

Mendon, Utah 84325

http://www.jd-biz.com/

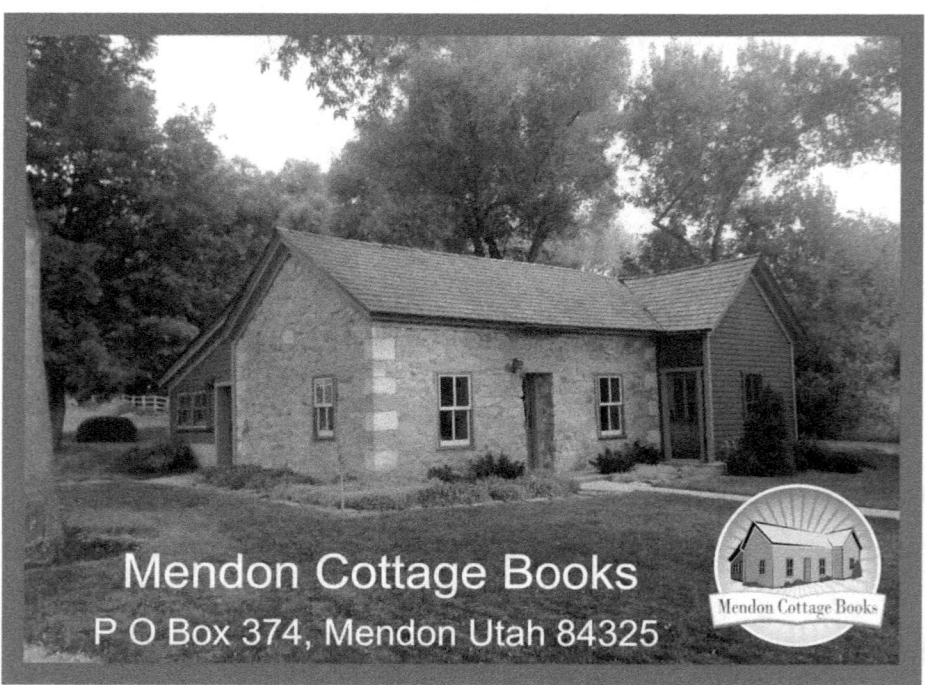